Why this book?

- Are you struggling to lose weight?

- Have you tried diets before but given up?

- Are you concerned about the long-term health implications of being bigger than you want to be?

If so, this book is for you. This is not another "get slim by next Friday" wonder cure. You may have tried those – they don't work and are not sustainable. This book will give you the facts. It will help you to:

- understand why you put on weight

- find a diet and exercise plan that suits you and your lifestyle

- lose weight slowly and sustainably – and keep it off.

This book has all you need to know for a new slimmer and healthier you!

First Steps out of Weight Problems

Catherine Francis

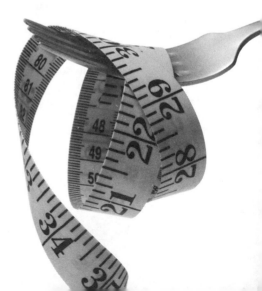

LION

All advice given is for information only and
should not be treated as a substitute for expert
guidance

Copyright © 2012 Catherine Francis
This edition copyright © 2012 Lion Hudson

The author asserts the moral right
to be identified as the author of this work

A Lion Book
an imprint of
Lion Hudson plc
Wilkinson House, Jordan Hill Road,
Oxford OX2 8DR, England
www.lionhudson.com
ISBN 978 0 7459 5538 4

Distributed by:
UK: Marston Book Services, PO Box 269,
Abingdon, Oxon OX14 4YN
USA: Trafalgar Square Publishing,
814 N. Franklin Street, Chicago, IL 60610
USA Christian Market: Kregel Publications,
PO Box 2607, Grand Rapids, Michigan 49501

First edition 2012
10 9 8 7 6 5 4 3 2 1 0

A catalogue record for this book is available
from the British Library

Typeset in 10/13 ITC Stone Serif
Printed and bound in Malta

Contents

Introduction

Are you worried you have a weight problem? Have your friends, family, or doctor expressed concerns about whether your size is affecting your health? Is it damaging your confidence, self-esteem, and happiness? Perhaps you've tried to slim down many times in the past and are losing hope you'll ever succeed.

If so, you're not alone. More than half of us are now overweight. Carrying excess pounds can dramatically affect your health and quality of life, and even shorten your life expectancy. However, you're not condemned to stay that way for ever. Armed with a little knowledge and determination, you can get back to a healthy size – and stay that way.

Back to basics

Obesity has become big business. A glance at the slimming section of your local bookshop may leave you bewildered by all the different diets and exercise plans on offer, each claiming to hold the key to effortless weight loss. Add to that countless advertisements for diet pills, meal replacements, and slimming clubs, and it's easy to be overwhelmed and feel like giving up before you start.

This book is designed to take you back to basics. Forget the gimmicks, fads, and trendy diets. This beginner's guide will explain the simple facts of how you've gained the unwanted pounds – and how you can lose them again,

 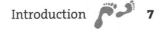

through easy changes to your diet and activity levels. It will guide you, step by step, through losing the weight healthily and sensibly, in a way that suits your lifestyle.

It's time to take charge

By understanding how your body works, you can take control of your size. This book will help you calculate how much weight you really need to lose (or perhaps why you don't need to lose any at all). You'll learn how to work with your body to whittle away the extra fat and reach your ideal size. Not every suggestion will work for you, because you're an individual – you can pick and choose the methods that suit you best.

Beating a weight problem is never easy – it takes commitment, and from time to time you'll fall off the wagon. So look out for lots of practical, tried and tested strategies to boost your motivation and keep you on track. There are also tips to boost your body's ability to release fat stores more efficiently, and once you reach your ideal size, you'll have the tools to keep the weight off for good.

There are also encouraging stories from fellow slimmers who've beaten their diet demons and are now enjoying a new healthy life. If they can do it, so can you!

Weights are given in stones/pounds and kilograms. A conversion table for stones to pounds can be found at the back of the book.

Dress sizes are UK sizes. A conversion chart for USA/Canada and Australia/New Zealand is included at the back of the book.

1

Do you need to lose weight?

If you're overweight, you're not alone. Here in the Western world, we're currently undergoing an "obesity epidemic". In the UK, more than half of adults are overweight, and a fifth are obese – that's nearly tripled since 1980. In the USA and Australia, the situation is even worse – over 60 per cent of the adult population are overweight, and over a quarter obese. Weight problems are also on the increase in children. Even our pets are developing weight-related health issues!

Being oversized isn't something you should feel guilty or ashamed about, as modern lifestyles make it very easy to pile on the pounds. However, carrying excess weight can dramatically affect your health, quality of life, and self-esteem. In fact, obesity is now one of the leading preventable causes of premature death. So congratulations on deciding to take action and tackle your weight problem.

Only greedy, lazy people are overweight.
As mammals, we're programmed to eat and gain weight
when possible, to get us through famines and leaner times.
However, in our modern Western world, food shortages
are rare, and the constant supply of high-calorie, high-
fat foods, combined with increasingly inactive lives, can
easily lead to weight problems.

Why should you lose weight?
Your motive for shedding the excess pounds may be more
about how you look than how you feel. It's certainly true
that slimming down can do wonders for your confidence
and self-esteem. However, perhaps more importantly,
maintaining a healthy size has countless benefits for your
health and quality of life. If you're overweight or obese,
getting back into your recommended weight range can:

• lower your risk of heart disease, high blood pressure,
  stroke, type 2 diabetes, and high cholesterol. Men are
  particularly at risk of cardiovascular diseases, because
  of where they tend to carry fat on their bodies. If
  you already have these conditions, losing weight can
  improve them, and you may be able to lower your dose
  of medication or even stop taking it altogether;

• reduce your likelihood of developing kidney disease,
  gout, gallstones, fatty liver, and certain cancers,
  including breast, womb, and colon cancer;

• improve your mobility and lower your risk of
  osteoarthritis, back and joint problems, and your

likelihood of needing a hip or knee replacement later in life;

- boost your energy levels and make it easier to be active without becoming exhausted and short of breath. You may also sweat less;

- improve your sleeping patterns and reduce sleep apnoea (when disturbed breathing wakes you regularly throughout the night, leaving you exhausted during the day). Losing weight can also reduce snoring (your partner will thank you for that!);

- boost your libido and improve your sex life;

- reduce your risk of stress incontinence (leaking urine when you laugh or cough);

- improve fertility (in both men and women) and boost your chances of conceiving. For women, being a healthy weight will help regulate your menstrual cycle and, if you become pregnant, lower your risk of having pre-eclampsia, birth complications, or a Caesarean section.

Even losing a modest amount of weight can significantly improve your health and well-being and add years to your life expectancy. So, what are you waiting for?

What people say...
At 17st 4lb (110kg), I found my job as a junior school teacher a real struggle. I had no energy and was often breathless. I suffered joint pain. I was going to the toilet several times a night and my doctor warned me I was in danger of developing type 2 diabetes. Taking out a pen and paper, I wrote a list of

reasons for wanting to be slim, such as improving my health, being able to run up the stairs without feeling ill, regaining my self-respect, and being able to wear nice clothes. Seeing my thoughts in black and white gave me the incentive I needed to get started on my weight loss plan.

Maggie, 28, now 9st 2lb (58kg) and size UK12

Over to you!

Like Maggie (above), take a few minutes to write down all the reasons you want to lose weight. Include current and potential health concerns, being happier with how you look, improving how you feel about yourself, and how being a healthier size may enhance your working life, relationships, and quality of life. Are you ready to tackle your weight problem, once and for all?

How much weight should you lose?

Perhaps you've been told by your doctor to lose weight for your health. Maybe family and friends say they're concerned about your size. Or maybe you're simply sick of not liking what you see in the mirror and finding it difficult to do the things you want.

On the other hand, women are constantly confronted by images of ultra-skinny celebrities and models in magazines, TV, and advertising, and men are also increasingly under pressure to achieve a gym-honed six-pack. This can lead to unrealistic expectations of what's "normal" and many of us believe ourselves to be "fat" when we're nothing of the sort. This can contribute to eating disorders such as anorexia and bulimia, and problems such as body dysmorphia, where people see themselves differently to how they truly are.

So, first of all, let's work out how overweight you really are, and how much you should aim to lose. There are several ways to do this.

Body Mass Index

People are different heights and builds, so simply weighing yourself doesn't tell you if you're overweight. The Body Mass Index (BMI) is a measure of your weight related to your height, and it's used by health professionals to assess whether your weight is putting your health at risk. There are BMI calculators available on the internet (in metric and imperial), but if you want to work it out yourself, here's how:

Divide your weight in kilograms by the square of your height in metres. So, for example, if you weigh 70kg and are 1.75m tall, your BMI is 70 ÷ (1.75 x 1.75), which gives a BMI of 22.9.

Here's how to interpret your BMI (for adults):

- Less than 16.5: severely underweight

- 16.5–18.5: underweight

- 18.5–25: healthy weight

- 25–30: overweight

- 30–40: obese

- More than 40: morbidly obese (meaning you are at risk of potentially life-threatening health problems).

Although the BMI index is helpful, it's only a guide, and every individual is different. For instance, serious exercisers are often heavier because they have a high muscle density (muscle weighs more than fat). Therefore, they may have a high BMI, despite being lean and healthy. This BMI index does not apply to children or pregnant women.

Find your weight range the easy way

If working out your BMI seems a bit complicated, don't worry – we've done the hard work for you. Find your height and weight on the graph opposite to see which weight category you're in, and the healthy range you need to aim for.

Waist measurements

Where you store fat on your body (partly controlled by genetics and gender) also makes a difference to your health. Carrying too much fat around your middle increases your risk of conditions such as heart disease, high blood pressure, type 2 diabetes, and some cancers. So whip out the tape measure and wrap it around your waist.

You have a higher risk of health problems if your waist is:

- more than 31½ inches (80cm) for a woman

- more than 37 inches (94cm) for a man.

The health risk increases further if your waist is:

- more than 34½ inches (88cm) for a woman

- more than 40 inches (102cm) for a man.

 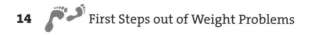

Weight in kilograms

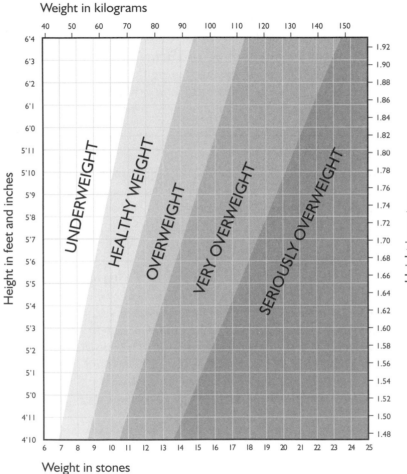

Height in feet and inches

Height in metres

Weight in stones

UNDERWEIGHT

HEALTHY WEIGHT

OVERWEIGHT

VERY OVERWEIGHT

SERIOUSLY OVERWEIGHT

Do you need to lose weight? **15**

Body fat percentage

The fitter and leaner you are, the lower your body fat percentage will be. A body fat monitor sends an electronic signal through your body, which passes through lean body tissue but meets resistance in fatty tissue. Some bathroom scales include a fat monitor, and many gyms have them on site. Women naturally carry more fat than men. Around 18–31 per cent is a healthy body fat percentage for women, compared to 10–25 per cent for men.

Over to you!

Use a BMI calculator or the handy graph on page 15 to work out what weight range you're in. Then check what your healthy range should be. This will give you an idea of how much weight you should be aiming to lose.

What people say...

My husband Carl didn't mind what size I was, but at 16st 3lb (103kg) I felt so unattractive I couldn't believe he was attracted to me, so our sex life suffered. I felt like a fat, sweaty blob compared to all his friends' wives, and was embarrassed for Carl having to put up with me on his arm. He insisted I looked lovely, but I couldn't accept he meant it. Now, I feel much better about myself, and our relationship has improved.

Andrea, 42, now 10st 2lb (64kg) and size UK12

If you're underweight

If you have a BMI of less than 18.5, you have an increased risk of conditions including osteoporosis (brittle bones), anaemia (iron deficiency), low resistance to infection, impotence in men, and amenorrhoea (absence of periods) in women. In this case, you should talk to your doctor about gaining weight.

If you're underweight or in your healthy weight range but still feel a compulsion to lose weight, consider whether you may have an eating disorder. Have your family and friends expressed concerns about your relationship with food and your body image? If so, please speak to your doctor. There is also a book in this series called *First Steps out of Eating Disorders* – see the **Useful resources** section at the back of this book.

When NOT to lose weight

If you're pregnant

Never go on a weight-loss plan if you're pregnant, unless specifically instructed to do so by your doctor. Your calorie requirement goes up slightly during pregnancy to cater for your growing baby and to sustain your body. It's natural to gain some weight during pregnancy, and there's plenty of time to lose it after your baby is born. But don't use pregnancy as an excuse to pig out on fatty, sugary foods – "eating for two" means twice as healthy, not twice as much! Eat a wholesome, varied diet for all the nutrients you and your baby need. Once you've given birth, don't start a diet or exercise programme until you've been given the all-clear by your doctor, midwife, or health visitor.

If you're breastfeeding

Again, breastfeeding means your body is working hard to produce nutritious milk for your baby, so don't limit your food intake. You may find you naturally lose weight while breastfeeding, but concentrate on eating a healthy, varied diet to sustain you and your baby. Taking some gentle exercise won't hurt, though.

During or after a major illness

If you're dealing with a major illness, or recuperating after one, concentrate on feeding yourself nourishing foods and getting plenty of rest to build up your immunity and recover your strength. Even during a mild illness, such as a cold or viral infection, it's best to give your body a rest from exercise. Once you're feeling strong again, you can turn your attention to your weight problem.

After surgery

If you've had an operation – including a Caesarean – it will take your body a while to fully recover. Gentle exercise such as walking or swimming may be fine, but get the go-ahead from your doctor before starting any exercise programme.

Dieting while on medication

If you're taking certain medications, such as some psychiatric drugs or insulin for diabetes, your daily dose may be calculated in relation to your body mass, or based on how much you normally eat. If you have any doubts, speak to your doctor before starting a weight-loss programme, and liaise with them regularly to reassess your dose as your weight changes.

 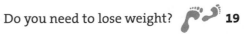

2

Why are you overweight?

People often wonder how they've managed to become overweight. But you only need to consume around 3,500 calories more than you burn to gain one pound (0.5kg). Put on a pound a month and by the end of the year you'll be nearly a stone (6kg) heavier. Give it five years and... well, you do the maths!

In the West, our weight is on the increase, and it's mostly down to changing lifestyles, some of which we're not even aware of.

Bigger portions

According to nutritional consultant Dr Lisa Young, the average portion sizes for meals, snacks, and drinks in the US have doubled or even tripled since the 1960s. In the UK, portions aren't quite as big (yet), but they have increased considerably, even in the last twenty years.

Relying on ready meals

Thirty years ago, people cooked most of their meals from scratch. Now, many of us are so busy we rely on ready meals, takeaways, and fast food. Unfortunately, these foods tend to be high in fat, sugar, and salt, all of which contribute to our bulging waistlines.

Eating on the run

Another consequence of our time-poor lives is that we're more likely to "graze" during the day – snacking and eating on the run instead of sitting down to three healthy meals. Without realizing it, we consume more calories that way, especially if the snacks we rely on are high in sugar and fat, as they don't keep us satisfied for long. It doesn't help that if you're looking to buy something healthy to eat on the run, snacks that aren't laden with fat and sugar are hard to find – even those healthy-looking cereal bars are often loaded with both.

A life sitting down

As our working environments become more automated, more of us spend our nine-to-five sitting behind a desk. Our leisure time also often revolves around passive activities such as watching TV or playing computer games – the average Briton watches twenty-six hours of TV a week. The less active we are, the less energy we burn – and those leftover calories are stored as fat. Improved technology means we're also less active in our daily lives. If you always drive instead of walking, take the lift rather than the stairs, and employ someone to do the housework, it's the perfect recipe for piling on the pounds.

Hidden calories

Many of us have no idea how many calories we're consuming in processed foods and even drinks. For instance, a large glass of red wine can contain over 200 calories – that's 10 per cent of your suggested daily calorie intake. A large latte can contain over 300 calories and almost a third of your recommended fat intake. Suddenly, your weight gain starts to make sense...

Slowing down with age

With each passing decade, your metabolism (the rate at which your body burns energy) slows down, particularly after the age of forty. That means you need to either lower your energy intake or increase your activity levels. Otherwise, the pounds will creep on – and they're harder to lose too.

What people say...

I started gaining weight after I got my first job. Several nights a week, I'd go to the pub with my workmates and drink four or five pints of beer, followed by pizza or chips. I didn't care too much when the pounds started to creep on – although when my first child was born, I realized it was hard to run around after him. But with a young family and a busy life, it was easy to fall back on convenience foods and takeaways. By my late 30s, I weighed over 17st (108kg) and couldn't walk up the stairs without feeling exhausted.
Barry, 44, now 12st 8lb (80kg)

Over to you!

Take a long, hard look at your lifestyle. Do you rely on ready meals instead of cooking meals from fresh ingredients? How active are you on a daily basis? Do you tell yourself you don't eat much, but nibble all day and down several drinks in the evening? Jot down all the aspects of your life that have contributed to your weight problem.

The excuses we use

It's all too easy to come up with excuses for being overweight. But if you hide behind those fat fibs, you'll never slim down.

- *"It's my genes."* It's true there is a gene linked to obesity, but inheriting it only makes you more susceptible to putting on weight. It doesn't make it inevitable. An active life dramatically reduces the effects of any genetic influence.

- *"I'm big boned."* Around 20 per cent of people have a larger frame, but they tend to be tall and muscular – and this won't make more than about a 10lb (4.5kg) difference to your weight.

- *"I've got a slow metabolism."* Being overweight is rarely caused by a slow metabolism, unless you have a medical problem. The truth is that being active boosts your metabolism, while being sedentary keeps it slower.

What people say...

As a child, I loved all the wrong foods – chocolate, pasties, and chips. By my sixteenth birthday, I weighed over 13st (82kg), but I believed it was "just the way I was". As an adult, I never ate fruit, only saw vegetables at Sunday dinner, and had ready meals or takeaways every evening. By the age of twenty-five, I weighed 19st (121kg) and was a size UK28 – yet I still convinced myself I was just "big boned".

Belinda, 34, now 9st 2lb (58kg) and size UK10

Emotional eating

Our relationship with food is often very emotional. Many of us comfort-eat when we feel lonely, unloved, stressed, or bored. If we have low self-esteem, we may not prioritize our own health or think we "deserve" to look and feel our best.

Many of us also learned habits and beliefs about food as children. We may have been taught to clean our plates, or told "waste not, want not". Sweet foods may have been used as a reward. These beliefs can influence our habits as adults, leading us to finish up the kids' leftovers rather than throw them away, or "treat" ourselves with favourite foods after a hard day.

In extreme cases, our relationship with food can lead to bingeing cycles or an eating disorder. If you're concerned you may have a problem, speak to your doctor. As already mentioned, there's also a book in this series called *First Steps out of Eating Disorders* – see the **Useful resources** section at the back of this book.

Over to you!

Consider how you feel about food. Do you eat to make yourself feel happier? Do you find it impossible to throw food away? Jot down how your experiences as a child may have contributed to your weight struggle.

Why have your previous diets failed?

Many people have tried (and failed) to shed the extra pounds many times over the years. Why do we get caught in the yo-yo dieting trap, losing weight over a few weeks or months, only to give up and pile it all back on again?

You take an all-or-nothing approach
If you're a perfectionist, a single slip-up may be enough to end your diet. You eat a biscuit, decide you've ruined your diet, and before you know it you're back to your old ways.

You crash-diet
If you slash calories and feel hungry all day, you won't be able to last long. Plus your body will think you're starving and will slow down your metabolism to compensate. You can't lose a stone (6kg) in a week, but take it steadily and you can lose a stone in two months.

You don't exercise
It's possible to lose weight from dieting alone, but it's much harder and takes longer. Exercise makes all the difference to seeing the fat melt away. Get fitter and your body burns energy more quickly, even when you're asleep.

You weigh yourself too often
Weigh yourself every day and you'll soon become demoralized by the scales not moving much (or at all), or even seeing small gains due to natural daily fluctuations. Get on the scales no more than once a week and you'll be encouraged by steady, measurable loss.

I was always embarking on the latest fad diet or joining another slimming club. I'd shed some weight, then lose motivation and slip back into my old routine. I'd put the weight back on – and more. Sometimes I did well – I got down to a size UK14 for my wedding. But I was soon back up to a size UK20 because it was a temporary fix and I didn't change my lifestyle.
Vicky, 47, now 9st 3lb (59kg) and size UK12

Why does weight always go on certain parts of my body?

Whether we're overweight or not, we all have a natural body shape and certain areas where we lay down fat. For instance, you may have heard women being described as "apples" or "pears". On pear-shaped women, fat gathers on the hips and thighs. Apple-shaped women carry fat on their tummies and waists. Men also tend to carry weight on their torsos.

Could a medical problem be causing your weight gain?

Obesity rarely has a medical cause, but there are some conditions that lead to weight gain. If you've put on weight without changing your lifestyle, and recognize the following symptoms, see your doctor.

Underactive thyroid
The thyroid is a gland in your neck that regulates metabolism. Having an underactive thyroid

(hypothyroidism) can lead to weight gain, and if it's not accurately treated with a replacement hormone, losing weight is very difficult. Other symptoms include brittle hair and nails, dry skin, fatigue, constipation, and a tendency to feel cold.

Hormone imbalance

Hormonal problems can lead to difficulties in burning off fat. For instance, polycystic ovary syndrome (PCOS) often goes undiagnosed, and can trigger a weight increase. Other symptoms include fertility problems, thinning hair, acne, irregular periods, and excess facial hair.

Cushing's syndrome is caused by an excess of the hormone cortisol. Fat accumulates around the face, torso, and back, while limbs remain slender. Other symptoms include muscle weakness, thin skin that bruises easily, poor wound healing, and hair loss in women.

Water retention

This doesn't normally amount to more than a couple of extra pounds (1kg) on the scales. However, if you quickly gain a large amount of puffy weight, see your doctor urgently, as excessive water retention can be a sign of heart or kidney failure. Other symptoms include shortness of breath, decreased urine output, loss of appetite, and fatigue.

Depression

People tend to eat stodgier foods and are less active when they're depressed, leading to weight gain.

Certain medications

Some people put on weight when they're taking drugs such as antidepressants, steroids, or the contraceptive pill. If you've struggled to fit into your clothes since starting a new medication, ask your doctor about alternatives, but don't stop taking it without medical guidance.

A tumour or growth

In extremely rare cases, extra weight can be caused by a large tumour or cyst. If you notice a rapid increase in a particular area of your body such as your belly, and have other symptoms, see your doctor.

What about sudden weight loss?

Unexplained weight loss can also be a sign of a serious illness. If the pounds are dropping off for no apparent reason, don't ignore it – get it checked out as soon as possible.

Over to you!

If you have concerns about any medical problems, book an appointment with your doctor. While you're there, ask them to take your blood pressure and do other general health checks. Explain you're planning to start a diet and exercise plan. They'll be delighted you're taking control of your health. Ask if they have any particular guidance for you, especially if you are obese or have any existing medical conditions.

3

How weight loss really works

We all wish we knew the secret to effortless slimming. When you scan the weight-loss section at your local bookshop, or the covers of magazines at the supermarket, it would appear that every expert believes they've discovered the key to shedding pounds painlessly – whether that's a particular food or food group, only eating at certain times of the day, or eating according to your blood type or body shape. On top of that, advertisers relentlessly target us with "no effort" quick fixes such as diet pills, slimming patches, and meal replacements.

The bad news is that there's really no magic bullet for melting away excess pounds without changing your lifestyle and putting in some effort. The good news is that the formula for losing weight is actually quite simple – and if you follow it, you can steadily whittle away the flab to reach your ideal size and stay that way.

The energy equation

Weight loss (and weight gain) is all about *Energy In vs Energy Out*. You take in energy (measured in calories) through food and drink. The food is broken down by your body and energy is released. This energy is then used to maintain all your basic bodily functions, from keeping your heart pumping to regulating your body temperature and using your brain. You also burn energy with every movement you make, from blinking to running a marathon.

You need to consume a certain number of calories a day just to keep your weight stable. This varies depending on your height and build, but for women the basic calorie requirement is around 2,000 a day, and for men it's around 2,500. If you consume more calories than you need, and you don't burn them off with exercise, the extra calories are stored as fat. Consume fewer calories than you burn and your body will release the energy stored in fat to make up the difference – and you'll lose weight. It really is that straightforward, and most successful diets, however they're packaged, boil down to the *Energy In vs Energy Out* equation.

There are, however, some ways to make losing weight easier, such as eating foods that release energy more slowly to keep you feeling fuller for longer, and types of exercise that burn fat more efficiently than others. You'll learn more about these in the following chapters.

I can "spot-reduce" fat on particular areas of my body.

Unfortunately, it's impossible to lose fat just from "problem" areas, such as upper arms or thighs. However, a healthy diet and exercise plan will whittle away excess weight all over your frame, which will improve your general shape. Plus, you can work on exercises to tone up muscles in certain areas, which will also help.

Say "no" to crash diets

The promise of swift weight loss is a tempting one. Shed 2st (13kg) in a month? Yes, please! But, actually, losing weight too quickly isn't good for your body and will make you more likely to regain it afterwards.

To get all the nutrients your body needs to stay healthy, you have to consume a certain number of calories a day. Take in fewer and your health will suffer. You will also be low in energy and will find it hard to function normally – you may find it difficult to think clearly, and become clumsy and prone to injury. Plus a very low-calorie plan is so tough to maintain that you'll soon give up and be back at square one.

Also, if your energy intake dips too low, your body will go into "starvation mode", and try to hold on to fat stores and lower your metabolism (the rate at which you burn energy) to preserve you through the "famine". When you start eating normally again, your body will lay down fat more quickly and you may end up heavier than you started.

Finally, crash diets don't re-educate your eating habits, so once the "diet" ends you are likely to fall back into old habits and the pounds will start creeping on again. So stay away from very low-calorie plans.

Mythbuster

Once I've lost the weight, I can go back to my normal life.

If, after losing weight, you go back to eating unhealthy foods and doing no exercise, you can expect to end up right back where you started – overweight and unhealthy. After all, that's how you got there in the first place. You need to see this as the start of a healthy new lifestyle – for ever! But that doesn't mean you can never have any fun. You can still enjoy your favourite treats in moderation.

What people say...
I was a classic yo-yo dieter. When a special occasion like a wedding was on the horizon, I'd go on a strict diet. Sometimes I'd lose a stone or more – but once it was over, I'd go back to my old ways and the weight would pile back on. Once, at 13st (83kg), I felt so desperate I tried a cabbage soup diet. I lost 10lb (4.5kg) in two weeks but it was revolting and I felt weak and ill. After a fortnight, I was scoffing crisps in relief, and my weight shot up to 13st 10lb (87kg). Eventually, I went on a sensible diet. It took a while to reach my target but it was painless – and the weight stayed off.
Sandra, 52, now 9st 10lb (62kg) and size UK12

Slow but steady wins the race

The best and most effective way to lose weight for good is to eat a healthy, varied diet of no fewer than 1,200 calories a day for women or 1,500 calories a day for men. Combine this with an exercise programme (at least thirty minutes of moderate activity, three to five times a week) to increase your energy output, and you'll see the fat slowly melting away.

You may lose as much as 7lb (3kg) in the first week, but this is mainly fluid loss. After that, you can expect to lose a steady 1–2lb (0.5–1kg) a week, which is a safe, healthy weight loss. You'll be able to maintain the plan and the weight is more likely to stay off. After reaching your target, you can gradually increase your calorie intake to maintain your new size.

Over to you!

Chances are you've tried and failed to slim down in the past, especially if you've gone on crash diets. Resolve now never to try a very low-calorie diet again, but instead to take a slow but steady approach that will boost your health and lead to successful, permanent weight loss. You know it makes sense!

What people say...

At the age of twenty, my weight of 14st 7lb (92kg) was already a health issue. My doctor told me my cholesterol and blood pressure were dangerously high and put me on medication. I devised a diet plan of 1,300 calories a day, and started walking with my baby in his buggy three times a week. I only lost 1lb or 2lb (0.5kg or 1kg) a week but I knew slow weight loss was healthy so I kept going. Just over a year later, I'd reached my goal.

Lindsay, 26, now 8st 4lb (53kg) and size UK10

Preparing to lose weight

The key to a successful slimming programme is to plan ahead. So before diving head first into a weight-loss regime, take some time to set your goal and decide how you're going to achieve it.

What's your target?

Most slimmers have a goal weight they want to reach (you can find your healthy weight range on the graph in Chapter 1). But it doesn't have to be about weight. Your target may be to get back into an item of clothing you love – you can check your progress by trying it on every couple of weeks. Or you may want to see your high blood pressure go down to a healthier level. It doesn't matter what your goal is, as long as you're clear about what you want to achieve.

Make a plan

If you start your diet and exercise regime without a clear strategy, you'll soon start to lose your focus and motivation. Of course, you may decide to make alterations to your plan as you go along, but you need to start with a clear understanding of your programme, so map it out and write it down.

Set a start date

Decide when your new lifestyle will begin. Choose a time when your stress levels will be low – not in the middle of a high-pressure work project when you'll be working long hours and eating on the run. Don't start a diet just before a holiday or big celebration with food and wine aplenty – you'll either fall straight off the wagon or feel miserable and deprived. A Monday may seem like the obvious day to start, but your initial enthusiasm may be waning by the weekend, when you'll be faced with negotiating family dinners, parties, or days out. Start on a Friday and you'll get through that first weekend while your motivation is still strong, setting you up for more successful weekends to follow.

Over to you!

Before you begin, read this book through to the end, making notes if it helps, so you understand all the principles of successful weight loss. Decide on your goal and how you'll measure it. Write it down and stick it somewhere you'll see it regularly. Write out a clear plan for your new, healthy diet, including weekly shopping lists. Think about what exercise you might enjoy and do some research, such as getting a timetable of local aerobics classes, signing up for tennis lessons, or putting together a walking programme. Nominate a date in your diary for your new lifestyle to begin.

4

Eating to lose weight

Let's turn our attention to the first half of the *Energy In vs Energy Out* equation. As you now know, there's no need to starve yourself to lose weight, especially if you're burning plenty of energy through exercise. But you do need to start controlling how much energy you take in through food and drink. That doesn't mean never enjoying your favourite treats, but it does mean learning to practise moderation. There are various ways to do this.

Calorie counting

Counting calories is a simple, scientific way of controlling your energy intake. A calorie (sometimes called a kilocalorie or kcal) is a measure of energy in food. To lose weight, you should aim to eat around 1,200 calories a day (women) or 1,500 calories a day (men). If you have a lot of weight to lose (over 3st/19kg), you can start on 1,750 (women) or 2,000 (men) calories a day, gradually decreasing your intake with every stone you lose. Most packaged foods are labelled with their calorie content, and a calorie guide will tell you what's in your basic ingredients and fresh foods.

Pros: It's an exact science – you can control exactly what you take in.

Cons: Weighing, measuring, and working out calories for every meal and snack can be time-consuming. (However, we've done some of the hard work for you in the next chapter, plus there are lots of calorie-counted recipe books available.)

Fat counting

We all tend to eat too much fat, which can have dire consequences for our health. So as well as managing your calories, it's a good idea to watch your fat intake. You should normally get no more than 33 per cent of your calories from fat. If you're trying to lose weight, aim for 25–30 per cent. That's a recommended 35g a day for women and 42g a day for men. Again, most packaged foods include the fat content on the label, and a calorie guide should provide fat information for the rest.

Pros: Limiting your fat intake will lower your risk of a host of health problems, including heart disease and stroke.

Cons: Low-fat doesn't necessarily mean low-calorie – many foods are fat-free but high in sugars.

Portion control

Some people don't have the patience for counting calories and fat grams, and prefer to practise portion control. This can be as simple as reducing your servings to half or three-quarters of what you normally eat. There are products that do the work for you, such as the Diet

Plate, which indicates the correct proportions of protein, carbohydrates, and vegetables in your meal. There are also other ways to measure portions – for example, a portion of carbohydrate should be the size of your fist, a serving of meat the size of a deck of cards, and so on (see the **Useful resources** section at the back for books and products).

Pros: Less time-consuming than working out calories, and more "portable" for different settings, such as the office canteen.

Cons: It's not an exact science and you may find your calorie intake slowly increasing without you realizing.

Slimming club "points"

Slimming clubs such as Weight Watchers and Slimming World have their own methods for measuring energy intake, revolving around points, "sins", and free foods. These are usually just a different way of counting calories and fat grams, but made simpler for members to follow.

Pros: Most of the hard work is done for you, although it still involves some weighing and counting.

Cons: May limit you to branded products and recipe books promoted by the club. You will need to join to access the resources.

Over to you!

Consider which of these methods will suit you best, and how much time and effort you're prepared to put into monitoring your energy intake. Invest in a pocket-sized calorie and fat guide you can refer to when shopping and cooking (see the **Useful resources** section at the back of this book). A calculator and kitchen scales may also come in handy.

 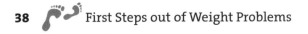

What people say...

At over 20st (127kg), I knew I had to take action. I wanted to design my own diet rather than follow one, so I bought a calorie guide and some kitchen scales, and started cooking. I stuck to 2,000 calories a day, with plenty of vegetables and fruit. I cut back on alcohol, but twice a week I allowed myself a chocolate treat. I even devised a spreadsheet to plot my calorie and fat intake against my weight loss.

Ricky, 37, now 12st 10lb (81kg)

Feed your body

A healthy diet isn't just about how many calories you consume – it's also about how you "spend" those calories. Of course, you could get your 1,200/1,500 calories a day from junk food and sugary snacks – but what's the point in being slim if you look and feel lousy, with a bad complexion and no energy to enjoy life? It's vital to nourish your body if you want it to function efficiently, especially if you're planning to exercise. So here's a quick crash course in basic nutrition.

Carbohydrates

These are broken down by your body to provide instant energy. They're found in starchy foods such as bread, pasta, cereals, rice, and potatoes, plus other fruits and vegetables. Wholegrain and brown varieties also provide plenty of fibre, which is needed for healthy digestion. Around 40 per cent of your calories should come from carbohydrates, but some types are better for you than others, as explained later in this chapter.

Proteins

Protein also provides energy and is essential for the growth and repair of body tissues. Muscles are made of protein. It's found in meat, fish, eggs, dairy products (also an important source of calcium), beans, Quorn, soya, pulses, and nuts. Protein should make up around 30 per cent of your calorie intake.

Fats

Fats help your body to function properly and aid the transport of nutrients around the body. They should make up no more than around 30 per cent of your calorie intake, but most of us eat far too much fat, leading to various health concerns. Choose unsaturated (good) fats such as nuts, seeds, avocado, and olive oil, and avoid saturated (bad) fat in butter, pastries, cakes, fatty meats, and high-fat dairy products.

Vitamins and minerals

These are essential for many different body functions. Fruits and vegetables are rich in vitamins and minerals (and fibre). Aim to eat at least five portions a day for good health.

For a balanced diet, eat a wide variety of wholegrain starchy carbohydrates, lean proteins (remove skin from poultry and trim visible fat off meat), beans and pulses, low-fat dairy products, fruit, and vegetables. Avoid processed meats (burgers and sausages), ready meals, salty snacks (such as crisps), sugary foods and drinks (fizzy drinks, sweets, biscuits, cakes), and high-fat foods (fried foods, pastries, creamy sauces, fatty meats).

Vegetarians and vegans

If you avoid animal products for ethical or health reasons, you can still enjoy a varied diet – and it's often easier to lose weight, thanks to a lower intake of saturated fats. Make sure you eat enough protein in the form of beans and pulses, tofu, Quorn, TVP (textured vegetable protein), soya products, nuts, and seeds. Non-vegan sources include eggs and dairy products. You should also keep an eye on your levels of iron (found in dried fruits, wholegrains, nuts, and green leafy vegetables) and calcium (in green leafy vegetables and fortified products such as soya milk), which can be lower in a vegetarian or vegan diet.

Over to you!

Resolve now to "spend" your calories wisely – don't get your 1,200/1,500 calories from junk and processed foods. Familiarize yourself with the different food groups, and make up your mind to eat a healthy, balanced diet. You may want to invest in a cookbook with calorie- and fat-counted recipes.

Mythbuster

I can save up my calories for an evening blow-out.
When you eat is as important as what you eat. To keep your energy up during the day, and give your body a steady supply of nutrients, you should distribute your food intake throughout the day, ideally as three main meals and two healthy snacks. This will also keep hunger pangs

at bay and stop you reaching for the chocolate when you're flagging.

What are low-GI foods?

GI stands for "glycaemic index" (and GL for "glycaemic load"). This is the speed at which carbohydrates are broken down by your body and sugars released. High-GI foods, such as chocolate, biscuits, and white bread, break down quickly, giving you an instant energy boost, quickly followed by a slump. Low-GI foods, such as brown rice, porridge oats, and most vegetables, break down slowly, giving you a steady supply of energy and making you feel satisfied for longer. They also help maintain stable blood sugar and insulin levels, so aim to eat more low-GI foods. See the **Useful resources** section at the back of this book for further information.

How you cook matters

Cooking methods make all the difference to how healthy your food is. Frying in oil will up the fat content, while boiling can leach out vitamins and minerals. Baking, grilling, and steaming are the best ways to keep foods low-fat and nutritious.

I can never have my favourite treats again.

Of course you can! If chocolate, crisps, or a glass of wine is your idea of heaven, simply budget some of your calories so you can enjoy your favourite treats a couple of times a week. If most of your diet is healthy, there's nothing wrong with spending a few calories on something you love. It'll keep you happy – and your motivation strong.

What people say...

At my first slimming club weigh-in, I tipped the scales at 21st 1lb (134kg). My club leader showed me that the food I bought, how I cooked it, and the amounts I consumed were all wrong. Out went the butter, lard, and cooking oil – I started baking and grilling instead of frying. I began buying more fruit and veg, and fewer desserts, white breads, and fatty meats. I could still have my favourite fish and chips once a week, but before long I was really enjoying my healthier diet.

Cathy, 43, now 11st (70kg) and size UK14

 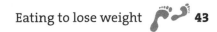

5

Making your diet work for you

Now you know how to eat to lose weight, it's time to apply it to real life. You may want to invest in some calorie-counted cookbooks and experiment with low-fat cookery. But for now, we'll give you a head start with some easy pick-and-mix meals.

This plan adds up to a daily intake of 1,200 calories. Each day, simply choose any breakfast (200 calories), lunch (300 calories), and dinner (400 calories), plus two snacks (100 calories each). We've given you seven of each to start you off. In addition, have half a pint of skimmed milk (100 calories) for drinks and cereals. You can swap the lunch and dinner if it suits you. Men and those starting on a higher calorie allowance (because you have more weight to lose) can add snacks accordingly.

Breakfasts

- Porridge made with 25g porridge oats and skimmed milk, topped with a sliced banana (and granulated sweetener if desired)

- 1 poached egg on 1 slice wholemeal toast with a smear of low-fat spread, plus an apple

- Large bowl of mixed fruits and berries with 1 small pot low-fat yogurt and a handful of mixed seeds

- 1 slice wholegrain toast topped with 2 grilled turkey rashers and grilled tomatoes

- Half a toasted bagel with 1 scrambled egg and 50g smoked salmon

- 40g low-sugar muesli with skimmed milk and a handful of blueberries

- 1 slice wholegrain toast topped with peanut butter, plus a pear

Lunches

- Sandwich made with 2 slices wholemeal bread, 30g chicken slices, salad, and a smear of light mayonnaise

- 50g of pasta with half a jar of tomato and basil sauce

- Any fresh or canned soup (up to 200 calories) and a wholemeal roll with low-fat spread

- Mushroom and pepper omelette made with 2 eggs and a sprinkling of grated cheese, and a salad

- Baked potato topped with cottage cheese, and a large salad

- Sandwich made with 2 slices wholemeal bread, 100g canned tuna, and mixed salad, plus a banana

- Ready-packed mixed-bean salad (up to 200 calories) and a wholemeal roll with low-fat spread

Dinners

- Large Greek salad made with 60g feta cheese, drizzled with oil-free dressing, and a wholemeal roll

- 150g roast chicken breast (skin removed) with 100g new potatoes, 2 servings of other vegetables of your choice, and low-fat gravy

- 150g salmon steak, grilled, with 50g brown rice and a large mixed salad

- Stir-fry made with 150g prawns, mixed vegetables of your choice, 1tbsp chilli sauce, and a small portion of wholewheat noodles

- 125g chopped turkey or 125g Quorn, mixed with 60g couscous, chopped cucumber, and spring onions, on a bed of salad

- 100g slice of roasted vegetable quiche with a large salad, plus an apple

- Small portion mushroom and bean pasta bake with unlimited green vegetables, plus a low-fat yogurt

Snacks

- A portion of any fruit
- 2 rice cakes, each topped with 1tsp peanut butter
- Tub of low-fat fromage frais
- 4 squares of dark chocolate
- Handful of cashew nuts
- Handful of vegetable crudités dipped in low-fat houmous
- 150ml glass dry white or red wine

Mythbuster

Coffee is calorie-free.
Black coffee contains no calories to speak of, but add full-fat milk, especially in lattes, or go for fancy varieties with chocolate, cream, and syrups, and the calorie count can be over 300. Choose filter coffee with skimmed or semi-skimmed milk, and go sugar-free or use sweetener instead.

Stay-on-track strategies
Eat regularly and you shouldn't feel hungry. But to make sticking to a healthy eating plan that bit easier, here are some tips to keep temptation at bay…

Plan ahead
The success of a diet is all in the planning. Decide on your menus for the week and shop accordingly. Know what you'll eat and when, and you're less likely to resort to snacks based on moods and cravings.

Remove temptation

If you know you can't resist a chocolate biscuit (or the whole packet), simply don't have them in the house. At the start of your diet, empty the kitchen of unhealthy foods that test your resolve – and never go food shopping on an empty stomach!

Stock up on healthy treats

Fill your fridge with healthy treats you can pick at when you get the urge. Fruits and berries are great for a sweet treat. Smoothies and fat-free yogurt are healthy and delicious. Nuts and seeds deliver a boost of "good" fats and are a valuable protein source. Low-fat houmous or avocado on rice cakes or crudités can meet a savoury craving.

Keep it varied

If you eat the same meals day in, day out, you'll soon get bored. Start trying different ingredients and make something new every week. Not only will it help side-step the boredom, it will also ensure you get a wide variety of nutrients in your diet.

Budget for treats

An austere diet will only make you miserable. Include a calorie allowance for your favourite indulgences a couple of times a week. You'll feel less deprived and it'll be easier to stick to your plan.

Over to you!

Before your weekly shop, make a meal plan for the next seven days and list all the ingredients you'll need – plus some healthy snacks such as fruit and nuts. Stick to your list and only buy what you need. Resolve to put one new thing in your shopping basket every week, such as an exotic fruit or vegetable you've never tried before. Keep your calorie guide with you in case you need to check anything.

What people say...

At 13st 10lb (87kg), I always felt unhealthy and exhausted. I started to control my calorie intake and portion sizes, cutting out takeaways and filling up on fresh fish, fruit, and loads of vegetables. If I wanted alcohol, I had the occasional vodka and slimline tonic. Strangely, I probably ate more than when I was overweight, but it was the right foods. I now feel full of energy and confidence.
Sandra, 46, now 10st (63kg) and size UK14

Simple food swaps

Still finding it hard to keep within your daily calorie allowance? Here are some easy food switches to slash calories and fat without even noticing:

- Swap full-fat milk for skimmed milk.

- Low-fat cheeses and yogurts are as tasty as full-fat, and are still rich in calcium.

- Choose pure natural juices and water instead of sugary squashes or fizzy drinks.

- Spirits are lower in calories than wine or beer.

- Swap creamy sauces for tomato-based ones, which contain very little fat.

- Choose plain boiled rice (ideally brown) instead of egg-fried or pilau rice.

- Scramble, boil, or poach eggs instead of frying.

- Have oven-baked potato wedges rather than chips.

- Sorbet is lower in calories than ice cream and contains almost no fat.

- Choose low-fat spreads, salad dressings, and mayonnaise.

Mythbuster

If it's labelled "low-fat", it must be healthy.
Low-fat products sometimes compensate for their lack of flavour with extra sugar. Don't automatically believe the packaging – check the nutritional label for yourself.

Don't become Cinderella
Occasions such as parties, drinks with friends, and family get-togethers can make sticking to your diet tough, but being on a healthy eating plan shouldn't spoil your social life. Here are some tricks for getting through those diet minefields:

- *At a wedding or party*, choose a table as far from the buffet as possible, so you're less likely to graze and go back for extra helpings. Load up your plate with salads, crudités and plain meats, and avoid the fried bites, pastries, and cheeses.

- *When out for drinks*, avoid sugary cocktails, wine, and beer, and go for spirits with slimline mixers instead. Alternate every alcoholic drink with a soft drink or water.

- *Before heading out*, eat a healthy snack containing protein and carbohydrates, such as egg on toast. It'll take the edge off your hunger and make you less likely to pick at nibbles and bar snacks.

- *If you're going to a restaurant*, see if you can check the menu online beforehand and work out the healthiest option. Once there, don't fill up on bread and butter. Ask for the dressing or sauce on the side. Have a starter or a dessert, but not both (or share one). Order wine by the glass, not the bottle.

- *Invited to a family dinner?* Offer to contribute a dish to the table, and keep it low-fat and healthy. Fill at least half your plate with vegetables.

What people say...

I was 12st 7lb (79kg) when I started my diet. I set myself a limit of 1,400 calories a day, and designed my own meal planner for meals and snacks. I started cooking all my meals from scratch – I didn't give up my favourite meals, I just made them fit my calorie allowance by using low-fat ingredients or eating smaller portions. I even took my calorie counter to restaurants.
Edie, 33, now 9st (57kg) and size UK10

6

Why exercise matters

The second half of the *Energy In vs Energy Out* equation involves burning off those excess calories and boosting your metabolism. As explained in Chapter 3, if you burn more calories than you take in, your body will break down its fat stores to release energy.

It's possible to slim through dieting alone – for instance, if you're disabled or have mobility problems. But if you're able to do some exercise several times a week, the weight will come off more readily. It will also develop your muscles, making you look more toned and improving your posture. It can even help stabilize your blood sugar levels, reducing those sugar cravings and making it easier to stick to a healthy diet.

If you consider a trip to the gym to be the stuff of nightmares, don't worry – in Chapter 7 you'll learn how to ease yourself into a fun, successful exercise programme that will suit you.

The benefits of getting fitter

As well as speeding up your weight loss and helping keep the flab at bay long-term, there are lots of advantages to getting fitter. Not convinced? Check out these benefits...

- *Less illness.* Exercise boosts your immune system, so you're less likely to succumb to colds and bugs. If you do catch something, chances are you won't feel as bad and you'll recover more quickly.

- *Improved sleep.* Regular exercise improves your quality of sleep. You'll find it easier to drop off and will wake feeling more refreshed.

- *Better brain power.* Working up a sweat boosts your mental agility. It may even help reverse the effects of ageing on the brain and lower your risk of dementia.

- *Feeling happier.* Exercise releases feel-good hormones serotonin and endorphins, which combat stress and have a positive effect on your mood. Keeping fit has been proven to help people suffering from depression.

- *Better skin.* Improved blood flow to the skin helps to deliver nutrients and remove waste matter, making your complexion clearer and more glowing.

- *More energy.* The more active you are, the more energy you'll have. Use it or lose it!

- *Living longer.* Exercise plays a major role in lowering your risk of serious diseases, including colon and prostate cancer and heart disease.

What people say...

At 13st 9lb (87kg), I hated what I saw in the mirror. I'd also had post-natal depression, which had developed into a long-term problem. I'd never felt lower. My doctor suggested I try to lose weight and get fit. I got an old exercise bike from my mother-in-law and began using it three times a week. I hadn't exercised for years but I was soon hooked and upgraded it for a cross-trainer. I also started swimming twice a week. Two years on, I feel like a different woman. I'm healthier, my skin is glowing, and my depression has lifted. My husband says it's like having a new wife.

Zeta, 34, now 9st 5lb (60kg) and size UK12

Three types of exercise

To get the full benefits, your workout should include three kinds of exercise – and, ideally, you'd do them in this order.

Cardiovascular exercise

"Cardio" is exercise that raises your heart rate and makes you breathe harder. It's sometimes called "aerobic" exercise, and it's great for your heart and lungs. It burns lots of calories and raises your metabolism, to help you lose weight. Cardio exercise includes running, cycling, dancing, aerobics classes, rowing, swimming – anything that gets your heart pumping. "High impact" describes exercise where both your feet leave the ground at the same time, such as running or skipping rope. "Low impact", where you're not pounding the ground – such as cycling or swimming – puts less strain on your joints, and is often a safer choice to start with if you're very overweight.

Resistance training

Also known as "strength training", this is any exercise that uses muscle contractions to build strength. This can mean working against outside resistance, such as free weights, elastic bands, or weights machines in the gym. Or it can involve working against your own body weight, such as press-ups, squats, and sit-ups. Swimming also offers resistance, as you have to work against the weight of the water. Resistance training builds muscle strength and density. It's helpful for weight loss because muscle is metabolically active, burning more calories than other body tissues, even at rest. So build those muscles and they'll keep burning calories, even when you're asleep! It will also make you look more toned.

Mythbuster

Weight training will make me bulk up.
Don't confuse weight training with weight lifting, power lifting, or bodybuilding. It takes serious dedication and hard work, using extremely heavy weights and a high-protein diet, to develop those large, bodybuilding muscles. You can't do it by accident! So, women, don't worry about developing an overly masculine physique – it won't happen.

Stretches

Stretching warm muscles after exercise is important, as it increases your flexibility and helps prevent injury and muscle soreness. It also helps you develop long, lean muscles to make you look slimmer. Do each stretch gently, holding it for about thirty seconds. Feel the stretch in the muscle, but don't overdo it to the point of pain. As time goes on, you'll be able to stretch further and become more flexible. A book or fitness instructor can explain specific stretches for the muscles you've used during your workout.

Can I target my problem zones?

As well as building muscle density, resistance training can help tone up particular areas that concern you. If you want a flatter tummy, sit-ups or crunches will help tighten your midriff. Hate your upper arms? Doing some lifts with free weights or machines in the gym will tone up the arm area.

Warming up and cooling down

It's vital to warm up at the start of a workout. This will raise your heart rate and body temperature, loosen your joints, and prepare your muscles for exercise. If you don't warm up, you're more susceptible to injury, such as pulling a muscle. So always spend the first five minutes doing something gentle, such as marching on the spot and circling your arms. Or try a slower version of whatever exercise you're doing – if you're using an exercise bike, cycle slowly and gently for the first few minutes.

Cooling down after your workout is also important. It allows your body to return to its normal resting state, making you less likely to feel sore or experience muscle fatigue afterwards. So, slow down the pace towards the end of your workout. This is also the time to do your stretches, while your muscles are still warm.

What people say...

When I signed up for a charity trek across Peru, I weighed 15st 3lb (97kg), and knew I'd have to get fit to manage the trek. I started exercising, building up to a forty-five-minute run in the morning and an hour's bike ride in the evening. I felt so good as the pounds fell off, it gave me the willpower to carry on. Eight months later, I'd lost 5st (32kg)! The trip to Peru was fantastic and I still get a huge buzz from exercise. My wife thinks I'm mad to get up early to go running, but it really sets me up for the day.

Simon, 53, now 10st 3lb (65kg)

The secret fat-buster

Although all exercise will help you burn calories and tone up, there's one technique that has been shown to burn fat faster than others. It's called "interval training" and it can apply to any form of cardio exercise.

Interval training simply means alternating between bursts of very intense exercise, which dramatically increases your heart rate, and periods at a slower, recovery pace. For example, if you're running or cycling, go as fast as you can for one or two minutes, then go at a slower pace (even walking) for three or four minutes. Follow this with another two minutes at maximum pace, then four at the slower pace, and so on.

Interval training has been shown to build fitness and burn fat faster than moderate exercise for the same length of time, probably due to the metabolism-boosting effects of the high-intensity intervals.

I should try to work out every day.
Even serious exercisers should take at least one day off a
week. This gives muscles an opportunity to rest and repair
themselves.

Over to you!

Are you ready to boost your activity levels and start exercising to aid your
weight loss? What other benefits would you like to get from working out?
Write a list of all the ways you'd profit from being fitter, such as having
better sleep and improved moods. Then turn to the next chapter to find out
how to create an exercise plan that will work for you.

7

Making exercise work for you

Now you know the theory, it's time to put it into practice. If the thought of hitting the gym brings you out in a cold sweat, or you currently find walking round the block a struggle, don't worry. There are activities out there that you'll enjoy and find it easy to stick to, and ways to gradually increase your activity levels – painlessly.

Find something you love

The most important thing is to find an activity you'll look forward to. If donning Lycra to leap about in an aerobics class is your idea of torture, or you go cold at the thought of exposing yourself in a swimsuit, don't force yourself. There are plenty of other activities that will raise your heart rate. Perhaps you've always fancied learning to dance? Would cycling to work – or for pleasure – appeal to you? How about skipping, hula-hooping, or Frisbee? Anything that raises your heart rate for thirty minutes several times a week will do.

Likewise, with resistance work, if you know you'll never stick to a weight-training plan, start thinking outside the box. A heavy gardening or DIY session can really work those muscles (you'll certainly feel it the next day). Hill walking is a great workout for legs. Or how about learning a new discipline such as Pilates?

Choosing your exercise is also about knowing yourself. Some people like to measure and plot their progress – in which case, gym equipment that tells you how far and how fast you've run or cycled is ideal. If you want to have fun while you get fit, Zumba classes, skating, martial arts, horse riding, or tennis might be the way to go.

Over to you!

Consider what you want to get from exercise. Do you like to measure your progress? Do you prefer to exercise alone or in a group? Are there any games or skills you've always wanted to learn? Make a list of the activities that appeal to you and do some research into local classes, clubs, or facilities. Resolve to try several different activities to find the ones you enjoy the most.

Starting out

Embarking on a new fitness regime can be daunting, especially if you haven't exercised for years (or ever). If you throw yourself straight into an hour-long, hardcore workout, you'll soon dread your exercise sessions and give up – plus you run the risk of injury. The key is to start gently and take it slowly.

 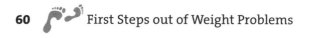

Get the OK from your doctor

If you have any health conditions, are very overweight, or haven't exercised for a long while, check in with your doctor first. They may advise you to steer clear of certain types of exercise.

Take it slowly

There's plenty of time to build up your fitness levels. If you're very unfit, walking is a great way to start. Set yourself the challenge of walking briskly for a couple of miles, three times a week. As it becomes easier, add another mile, then another. If you join a class, don't push yourself further than you're comfortable with. Listen to your body and rest when you need to – the instructor and other class members will understand.

Keep it low-impact

If you're very overweight, stick to low-impact exercise until you've slimmed down a bit. High-impact workouts such as running or skipping put a strain on your knees and ankles, and being heavier increases your risk of injury. Power walking, swimming, or cycling are easier on your joints.

Get professional advice

If you feel out of your depth, get some guidance from an expert. If you join a gym, there'll be instructors on hand to explain the equipment and suggest a programme for you. If you go to a class, have a chat with the teacher beforehand. They'll be able to give you some pointers and keep an eye on you to ensure you're doing the moves correctly.

What people say...

I was 12st 7lb (79kg) and feeling very unhealthy when my sister gave me her old bike. I hadn't cycled since I was ten years old, but I thought it might be fun. It was! Before long, I was cycling the eight-mile round trip to work. It gave me confidence, I had more energy, and my brain felt sharper too. I now cycle 100 miles (160km) a week, have joined a cycle club, and even did a 1,000-mile (1,600km) tour from Land's End to John O'Groats. It's my favourite pastime and I've made loads of friends through it, including my boyfriend.

Susan, 36, now 10st 7lb (67kg) and size UK14

Your fitness kit

There's plenty of fitness equipment you can invest in if you want to, from exercise bikes to weights machines to all manner of fancy sportswear. But if you're on a budget, there are only a few things you really need...

- *Loose, comfortable clothing.* Shorts or tracksuit bottoms and a vest or T-shirt will be adequate.

- *A good sports bra.* This is vital for women, especially if you're well endowed. Holding it all in place will keep you comfortable while you exercise. Go without a sports bra, and all that bouncing around may lead to sagging breasts.

- *Good trainers.* This is essential for exercise that involves any impact, especially running. If you don't wear well-fitting sports shoes with plenty of cushioning and bounce, you risk injury.

- *A bottle of water.* It's vital to keep well hydrated while you sweat, so drink plenty before, during, and after exercise.

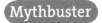

I can't afford to get fit.
Gym memberships and classes can take their toll on your bank balance, but there are lots of ways to get fit without spending much. Walking, running, and hiking cost nothing (except a decent pair of shoes). Buy a fitness DVD and you can use it at home as often as you want. Bottles of water or cans of food make good substitutes for hand weights. Being on a budget is no excuse not to get fit.

Stay-on-track strategies
It isn't always easy to stick to a fitness programme. When you have to fit it in between work and family responsibilities, your workout can be the first thing to go. Here are some tips to help keep you on track...

Put it in your diary
Treat your workouts as dates that can't be broken. If you just have a vague intention to do three workouts this week, it's easy to put them off when you're busy and tired, and then realize you haven't broken a sweat in a week. Schedule sessions in your diary, make it clear to others that you'll be busy, and don't cancel them unless absolutely necessary.

Keep it varied

As your body gets used to a certain exercise regime, your fitness and weight loss may plateau. The key is to keep changing it and challenging your body. Every six weeks or so, try something new, or change/increase something in your normal workout – run a bit further or add some weight to your resistance. Anything that keeps it interesting and moving forward.

Have a "fit buddy"

Research shows you're more likely to stick to a fitness schedule if you work out with a friend or partner. You can encourage each other to keep going. You can try pair sports such as badminton. If you arrange to meet your friend to go walking or running, it's harder to wriggle out of it if you're letting someone else down.

Set yourself goals

Having something to work towards will challenge you and keep you motivated. Currently walking three miles? Work towards walking four miles. Cycling at 10km an hour on an exercise bike? Try upping the gear for every other mile. If you're someone who thrives on a serious challenge, sign up for a sponsored 5km or 10km run, so you have to train for it.

Mythbuster

Personal trainers are only for the rich and famous.

A personal trainer may seem extravagant, but many people use them to get some extra help with designing their workout and staying motivated. They may be a pricey investment, but even seeing a personal trainer once every couple of months can help keep you on track and progressing.

Stay active every day

Being fit isn't just about gym sessions – it's about making your everyday life more active. So be on the lookout for ways to keep your body moving, especially if you work in a sedentary job. Here are a few ideas:

- Walk any trip of less than a mile rather than taking the car.

- Take the stairs instead of the lift or escalator.

- Go walking with a colleague during your lunch hour.

- Every hour, take a screen break from your computer to stretch and do a circuit of the office.

- Get off the bus one stop earlier and walk the rest of the way.

- Walk to a colleague's office to deliver a message rather than sending an email.

- March on the spot during every TV advert break.

- Park as far as possible from the exit in the car park.

What people say...
As a single mum, gym visits weren't practical for me. Instead, I started walking three miles to the shops pushing the buggy, rather than taking the bus. I took my daughter to the park for daily play sessions, which wore us both out! I also borrowed an

exercise bike and started using it at home after she was in bed. I weighed 11st 11lb (75kg) when I started. I'm now slim, fit, and confident, and when my daughter starts school, I'm going to join a daytime aerobics class.

Gemima, 24, now 8st 13lb (57kg) and size UK10

 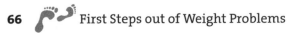

8

More ways to boost your weight loss

By now, you know there are no magic bullets when it comes to weight loss, and the simple equation of burning more energy through exercise than you take in as food and drink is the key to seeing the excess pounds melt away. However, there are some healthy habits that can boost your body's ability to function well and release fat stores more efficiently.

Never skip breakfast
We've all heard that breakfast is the most important meal of the day, but it's tempting to assume that if you skip brekkie, you can save a few calories and shed more weight. Wrong! Research shows that people who eat breakfast every day are less likely to be overweight than those who regularly start the day on an empty stomach.

That's because your metabolism slows down during the night to conserve energy and get you through the nightly "fast". You need to break that fast ("break-fast") to kick-start your metabolism again. Plus, if you don't fuel your body for the day, your energy levels will slump, and by mid-morning you'll find those fatty, sugary snacks almost impossible to resist.

Mythbuster

Cereal is the ideal breakfast.
Many cereals – even those marketed as healthy or for slimmers – are high in sugar. A blood sugar rush isn't a great way to start the day: by mid-morning, you'll get the corresponding slump and crave another injection of the sweet stuff. Wholegrain cereals with no added sugar or salt are a good choice, so select your cereal carefully. One containing nuts and seeds is even better, as it will provide protein. See Chapter 5 for other healthy breakfast choices.

Get your eight hours a night

Not getting enough sleep can increase your body's production of the hormone ghrelin (which triggers feelings of hunger) and decrease its production of leptin (which tells your brain when you're full). These combine to make you feel more hungry during the day. Lack of shut-eye can also play havoc with your insulin levels, leaving you craving sugary, energy-fix foods.

There's also some evidence to show that insufficient sleep can encourage your body to burn muscle rather than fat to release energy. This not only means you'll burn less body fat, but muscle loss will lead to a lower metabolism.

Research at the Obesity Research Center at Columbia University found that people who are sleep-deprived are 73 per cent more likely to have weight problems than those who get seven to nine hours' sleep a night. What better excuse for an early night?

Drink plenty of fluids

A well-hydrated body will function better, flush out waste products more efficiently, and allow itself to release fat from cells more easily. If you become dehydrated (and many of us are mildly dehydrated a lot of the time), your internal processes become more sluggish. You'll feel lower in energy too, so you're likely to be less active.

Aim to drink two litres (around eight large glasses) of fluid a day – more when you're exercising. That may sound a lot, but if you keep a drink on your desk and sip as you work, you'll soon down your quota. It will also improve your skin and boost your concentration levels. Plus we often think we're hungry when we're actually thirsty, so a drink can ease the urge to snack. Water is best, but low-sugar squash, diluted juices, tea, coffee, and herbal teas all count towards your daily intake.

What people say...
When my weight hit 12st 6lb (79kg), I realized I had to take action, so I embarked on a healthy diet plan. Whenever I felt hungry, I drank a glass of water before reaching for food. I was amazed by how frequently I'd been confusing hunger with thirst. I must have saved thousands of calories that way.
Debbie, 33, now 10st 3lb (65kg) and size UK14

Eat slowly

We're all guilty of bolting our food at times – sometimes we barely have time to taste it. However, eating too quickly isn't good for your digestion or your weight. Eating slowly and chewing food thoroughly allows your digestive enzymes to get to work, improving your digestion and absorption of nutrients. It also gives your brain time to register that your stomach is full (this can take around twenty minutes). Start to eat more slowly, savouring each bite and chewing it well.

Ease up on salt

We all need a small amount of salt in our diets, but too much is bad for our health, pushing up blood pressure and increasing the risk of stroke and heart disease. Although it doesn't contain any calories, a higher level of salt also leads to increased thirst and fluid retention as the body tries to maintain the correct concentration of electrolytes. Adults should consume no more than 6g of salt a day (that's around one teaspoonful), but most of us consume significantly more, so keep an eye on nutritional labels and avoid adding salt to meals. Try using a reduced-sodium salt alternative such as LoSalt, and experiment with herbs and spices to add flavour.

Mythbuster

I hardly eat any salt!
Unfortunately, salt finds its way into most processed foods – even basics like bread and baked beans. Levels in ready meals can be extremely unhealthy. Get into the habit of

choosing low-salt varieties, and checking the nutritional labels on food to spot that hidden salt.

Eat little and often

Many people trying to lose weight find eating little and often works best for them. It helps keep that all-important metabolism ticking over. Plus it keeps your blood sugar levels stable, which makes you less likely to experience an energy dip and reach for a sugary snack to give you a lift. So rather than three large meals a day, eat three small meals and two or three healthy snacks, leaving no longer than three hours between eating.

What people say...
At 13st 1lb (83kg) and rising, I was worried about my weight. But when I stopped snacking between meals, I ended up feeling tired and light-headed. Then I'd break and reach for a chocolate bar or a cola to pep me up. I discovered that snacking on low-GI foods such as oatcakes, nuts and seeds, porridge, and apples was great for regulating my energy levels and helping me feel more balanced. I soon stopped getting sugar cravings, my tiredness eased – and the weight dropped off.
Karen, 35, now 8st 10lb (55kg) and size UK8

Beat stress

During times of stress, your body produces cortisol, a hormone that urges you to eat. Cortisol increases your insulin production and your levels of glucose (sugar), which is then stored as fat. High levels of cortisol also make you more likely to store fat on your abdomen, as the fat cells there are more sensitive to the hormone. This not only adds to that muffin top or beer belly you're trying to lose, but is also linked with greater health risks (such as heart problems and diabetes) than when fat is stored on your bottom and thighs.

If you're constantly overwrought, try to find ways to de-stress. Delegate more at work, work off your frustration in the gym, try to eke out some "me time" at home for a relaxing bath – whatever helps you chill out and lower those stress levels.

Over to you!

All these tips are not only good for losing weight – they'll also help boost your general health. So start practising them right away in preparation for your slimming programme. If it seems like too many changes to make at once, just choose one healthy habit at a time to concentrate on, and as each one becomes a natural part of your daily routine, add another one. Re-read this chapter from time to time during your weight-loss challenge, as a reminder of the beneficial patterns you want to cultivate.

Do slimming aids work?

There are many products that claim to help you shed weight, from herbal supplements to "fat magnets" to tablets that swell in your stomach to fill you up. There's a limited amount of clinical evidence that some of these products can help speed up weight loss, but many have no research to back them up, and none will work on their own – you'll still need to improve your diet and activity levels to lose weight.

Many products have unpleasant side effects, such as excess gas, stomach pains, diarrhoea, or feeling hot and jittery. Some, such as fat binders, can hinder the absorption of fat-soluble nutrients including vitamins A and K. All in all, your best bet is to stick to a healthy diet and exercise plan, and perhaps take a general multivitamin and mineral supplement to ensure you're not deficient in any important nutrients.

Weight-loss surgery

Operations such as liposuction and gastric bands have gained a lot of publicity in recent years, and some high-profile celebrities have lost impressive amounts of weight with a gastric band.

It's true that some people find bariatric (weight-loss) surgery effective. But remember that, like all surgery, it comes with risks such as infection, accidental injury, blood clots, hernia, anaesthesia complications, and even death. Gastric bands, which limit how much food you can eat, can also lead to malnutrition (and associated health problems such as anaemia and osteoporosis), diarrhoea, constipation, gastric obstruction, nausea, ulcers, and gallstones.

If you're determined to have surgery, ask your doctor to recommend a specialist. Don't be tempted by a "surgery holiday" abroad – it may be cheaper but it may not be regulated to the same standards as in your own country. If something goes wrong, you won't have access to aftercare, or recourse to the disciplinary bodies that govern medical practice.

9

Maintaining your motivation

You now know how to lose weight slowly, steadily, and fairly painlessly. But, of course, we all know it's not that easy. Sticking to a diet when you're used to eating whatever you fancy, and disciplining yourself to exercise when you don't feel like it, is a tough challenge. Maintaining your resolve for months on end is no mean feat, especially if your weight loss plateaus for a while.

This is where we turn to your greatest weight-loss weapon: your mind. There are lots of ways to boost your motivation. Here are ten tried and tested strategies to help keep you on track during the tough times.

1. Set small goals
If you have several stones to lose, it's easy to feel overwhelmed by the task. Progress can seem so slow that

you lose the will to keep going. Divide your weight loss into small, achievable goals – say, half a stone (3kg) at a time. Celebrate each step on your way to your target. Perhaps even promise yourself a little reward for reaching each goal, such as a luxury bubble bath, tickets to a sports event, or a book you've been wanting to read.

What people say...
At 16st (102kg), I had a lot of weight to lose and it was coming off so slowly – 1lb or 2lb (0.5kg or 1kg) a week – that I wondered if I'd ever reach my target. So I started setting myself smaller goals: half a stone by my birthday; 3lb (1.5kg) in time for a party. It made it seem more achievable. Four months later, I'd lost 2st (13kg) and people started complimenting me. After fourteen months, I'd reached my ideal weight and felt fantastic.
Jenny, 25, now 10st 8lb (67kg) and size UK12

2. Keep a diet diary
Research shows that people who keep a record of everything they've eaten are more likely to stick to a diet, and consume fewer calories overall. Record each meal, snack, and drink, including every morsel you've grazed on during the day. Review it weekly – you may be surprised to find you're eating more than you thought. It will also help you see patterns developing, identify what's working best for you, or spot that your calorie intake has gradually increased without you noticing. If you also keep a record of your moods and feelings, it can be helpful for identifying emotional eating patterns. Turn to the back of the book for an example of a diet diary chart.

3. Plot your progress

There's nothing like seeing the weight come off to encourage you to keep going. Draw up a chart or graph on which to plot your weight loss each week. Stick it somewhere you'll see it, such as over your desk or on the fridge. When you have a disappointing week or start losing enthusiasm, a glance at the graph will remind you how far you've come. There's a chart at the back of the book you can use. You may prefer to keep a record of your vital measurements and how they're changing. Or perhaps take a photograph of yourself with every half-stone you lose and enjoy watching yourself shrink.

Mythbuster

I should weigh myself every day.
Your weight naturally fluctuates by a pound or two due to fluid retention and hormones. When the scales don't go down for a few days – or even go up – you may become demoralized and feel like giving up. But these daily fluctuations don't reflect your overall weight loss. Get on the scales no more than once a week for a reliable measure of your progress. Weigh yourself at the same time of the day – ideally first thing in the morning, before eating, and naked.

4. Have something to work towards

Motivation can come in the form of a special event on the horizon – a wedding, special party, or holiday where you'll be getting your body out on the beach. Work out how much weight you can realistically lose by the event and mark the date on your weight-loss chart so you have something to aim for. Keep reminding yourself why you want to lose the weight and how much more you'll enjoy the experience when you feel good about yourself.

5. Get people on side

Support from the people around you can make all the difference, so ask your friends, family, and partner to help. They can avoid putting food temptations in your path and encourage you to exercise when you're not in the mood. Even better, if you have a friend who also wants to shed the pounds, you can urge each other on when you're feeling discouraged.

But beware: not everyone wants you to lose weight. Some people may feel threatened by the idea of a confident new you. If you're aware of someone undermining your efforts or putting temptation in your path, it might be best to see less of them while you slim – or at least avoid eating with them – and keep your weight loss aims to yourself.

What people say...

My husband Ted was 20st 7lb (130kg) and I was 15st 3lb (97kg). We knew we both needed to tackle our weight problems, and we decided to do it together. Food shopping and saying "no" to our favourite sugary treats was tough, but we were determined, and with each other's support it became easier. We also went for long walks and cycle rides together. It was a joint project, and without each other's encouragement we'd never have lost so much weight.
Mandy, 46, now 10st 4lb (65kg) and size UK12 (Ted also lost over 5st/32kg)

6. Think positive

Instead of focusing on how unhappy you feel now, focus on how positive you'll feel when you achieve your goal. It will help to drive you towards your target. So instead of telling yourself, "I don't want to be fat and miserable" (which will simply reinforce your negative feelings), say to yourself, "Soon I'll be slim, confident and happy." You'll feel more encouraged to make it a reality. Likewise, don't stick up a "fat" photo of yourself to remind you of what you don't want to be. Instead, choose a photo of yourself when you were slim and healthy, to impress that image on your mind.

7. Don't keep your "big" clothes

As you move down the sizes, you'll soon be swamped by your current clothes. But if you bag them up and store them "just in case", you're subconsciously admitting you may regain the weight. If you're serious about slimming down this time, act as you mean to go on and get rid of clothes that are too big for you. Remind yourself you'll never need them again.

What people say...
I weighed nearly 17st (108kg) when I started. As the months went by, my dress size dropped rapidly. When my clothes became too big, I'd take them all to a local charity shop. While I was there, I'd stock up on clothes in the next size down, as I didn't want to spend a fortune on clothes when I was continuing to lose weight. In fifteen months, I went from a size UK28 to a size UK10 – and then I splashed out on a whole new wardrobe of gorgeous outfits!
Joanna, 49, now 8st 7lb (54kg) and size UK10

8. Join a slimming club

If you're someone who thrives on group support, a club such as Weight Watchers or Slimming World can be great for keeping you on track. Weekly weigh-ins and encouragement from your group leader and fellow members can give you an extra incentive for sticking to your plan. In most cases, you can keep going for free after you've hit your target, so the pounds don't creep back on – and you can encourage fellow slimmers with your success.

Mythbuster

Slimming clubs are humiliating.
Don't be fooled by how slimming clubs are portrayed on comedy shows. You'll be weighed in a discreet way and your weight won't be broadcast to everyone. You're unlikely to be the largest person there, and who can relate better to your struggle than others in the same boat? You'll get plenty of understanding and support.

9. Dress to impress

You may be waiting to reach your ideal weight before making an effort with your appearance. You may think, "What's the point in trying to look good and wearing nice clothes when I'm fat?" But looking your best will build your confidence and self-esteem, which in turn will boost your determination to reach your goal. Start dressing to flatter your shape, whatever your size. Pass over the dark, baggy tents – they only make you look bigger. Instead, choose fitted clothes in nice colours. Women, style your hair, wear make-up, and buy underwear with good support. Men, have your hair trimmed regularly, keep yourself groomed, and invest in some good aftershave. Before you know it, you'll have a spring in your step and will be feeling stronger and more able to persevere.

10. Visualize it

Visualizations may sound a bit hippy, but many people find them helpful for keeping their eyes on the prize. Spend a few minutes in bed at night imagining yourself as you want to be – slim, healthy, confident, feeling strong and good about yourself. See the image in as much detail as you can, and it will help you stay focused. Affirmations can also help. You may feel silly saying them out loud, but slogans like "I'm slim, happy, and in control" or "I'm not large, I'm in charge!" can help you say "no" when unhealthy cravings strike.

Oops, I fell off the wagon

It's inevitable that, sooner or later, you'll slip up. You may give in to temptation and end up bingeing on chocolate or crisps. You may have several drinks too many on a night out, and then find it impossible to pass the chip shop on the way home. Or, if you've got a perfectionist streak, just one biscuit could be enough to tip you over the edge, and you'll think, "Well, I've ruined my diet now – I might as well eat the rest of the packet, plus a family-size trifle for good measure!"

So be ready. If you slip up one day, simply put the matter behind you when you go to bed, and start afresh in the morning. Add in some extra exercise the next day if it makes you feel better. And remember: one spoiled day does not ruin a diet. But throwing in the towel altogether certainly will.

Over to you!

If your diets have failed in the past because you've slipped up and found it impossible to get back on track, resolve now never to let it happen again. Remind yourself you're not perfect and you *will* make mistakes, but it doesn't have to mean failure. Start gathering your motivational tools now, before you kick off your new lifestyle. Prepare your progress graph and diet diary, get family and friends on side, and start your visualizations.

 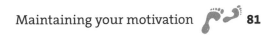

10

Keeping the weight off for good

If you want to stay slim this time, you can't view your diet and exercise programme as a temporary fix to be abandoned once you've lost the flab – you have to treat it as a permanent lifestyle change. If you go back to your old ways, the weight will creep back on and you'll have to start all over again.

However, once you've hit your target, you can afford to relax a little. In fact, you'll have to, otherwise your weight will continue to drop and you'll end up underweight. That's where a maintenance plan comes in.

Find your happy medium
Finding the *Energy In vs Energy Out* balance to maintain the size you've achieved through all your hard work is a process of trial and error. It's about discovering what

works for you as an individual. But you need to take it slowly. Increase your calorie intake too quickly and your body may react by storing the sudden increase of energy as fat.

Experts suggest adding around 200 calories to your daily allowance (through slightly bigger portions or healthy snacks) and monitoring your weight for a couple of weeks. If the weight continues to come off, add another 100–200 calories a day and see what happens. If your weight starts creeping up again, knock 100 calories off and continue to watch the scales. Eventually you'll find the calorie intake that keeps your weight steady. Continue to eat a varied diet with plenty of fruit and veg, healthy carbohydrates, and low-fat proteins, and you can't go far wrong.

Keep exercising

One of the keys to being able to eat well and not regain the weight is regular exercise. By burning off energy, keeping your metabolism working efficiently, and sustaining good muscle mass, you'll find you can be much more relaxed about what you eat. Stay active and your body will naturally maintain its weight, meaning you can enjoy your favourite treats (in moderation!) without paying the price on your waistline.

So, just because you've reached your target, don't give up working out. You may decide to do fewer sessions a week, if that suits you. But keep challenging your body and trying different kinds of activities to keep you interested. Continuing to exercise will also help keep your heart healthy and your blood pressure stable, and reduce your risk of numerous health problems.

Have a strategy ready

It's a good idea to keep monitoring your weight on a regular basis – perhaps every week or fortnight. You're only human, and sooner or later the scales may start to creep up again as you naturally pay less attention to your portion sizes, give in to the lure of the biscuit tin too often, and have less time to exercise, or as your metabolism naturally alters as you get older. It's much better to take action when just a few pounds have crept on than suddenly realize you've gained a stone and have a bigger challenge on your hands.

Have a strategy ready and you'll nip the problem in the bud before it gets out of control. Review your portion sizes or go back to keeping a food diary for a couple of weeks. Are you eating more than you realized? Think about your activity levels. Have you become more sedentary over time?

Start calorie counting again or go back to your tried and tested diet for a while to re-establish a healthy eating plan and pull your portion sizes back into line. Or try adding an extra weekly exercise session. You'll quickly get your weight under control again – before it starts controlling you.

What people say...
After losing over 4st (25kg) twice before, I was determined not to have to do it again. This time, instead of falling back into old habits, I continued eating healthily, checking my calorie intake from time to time and weighing myself every month. I also stayed active instead of slipping back into being a couch potato. I take our two dogs for long walks every day, and take my granddaughter swimming every week. I have loads of

energy and can easily run up the stairs to my third-floor office.
This time, I've kept the weight off for three years.
Sandy, 53, now 9st 10lb (62kg) and size UK12

Seven secrets of slim people

You're now a slim person – but it may take a while for you to catch up and start feeling and thinking like one. In the meantime, begin copying the behaviour of naturally slender people and you'll establish habits that will help keep you in good shape for life.

1. Always have breakfast

As explained in Chapter 8, studies show that people who regularly eat breakfast are more likely to be slim than those who skip the first meal of the day. If you're always in a rush in the morning, take a healthy breakfast to work to have at your desk – perhaps some low-sugar cereal and yogurt, or a pot of microwaveable porridge with a handful of seeds.

2. Only eat when you're hungry

In the Western world, food is so plentiful that many of us have lost touch with what it feels like to be physically hungry. On top of that, many of us crave foods for their flavour, an energy hit, emotional reasons, or simply habit and association. But naturally slim people only eat when they're physically hungry. So before you put something in your mouth, ask yourself: "Do I have that hollow feeling in my stomach that indicates my body wants food?" If you don't, leave it an hour and see how you feel.

3. Stop when you're satisfied

Start to eat more slowly and mindfully, enjoying each mouthful and giving your stomach time to communicate with your brain. Instead of eating until you're stuffed, or always clearing your plate as you may have been taught as a child, stop regularly to ask yourself: "Am I satisfied?" If you are, put down your knife and fork and don't keep eating for the sake of it.

4. Stay active

Being fit isn't just about working out. Naturally slim people tend to be more energetic in general. So practise choosing the active option. Use the stairs instead of the lift. Walk rather than take the car. Take the kids to the park on a Sunday afternoon instead of sitting in front of the TV. Every action will help to keep your metabolism ticking over.

5. See food as fuel

If you tend to eat when you're sad, lonely, or bored, find other ways to fill the void. Naturally slim people don't tend to have a strong relationship between feelings and food. They see food as a pleasure and a fuel – not a reward, punishment, or comfort. Look for other ways to deal with your emotions.

6. Sit at the table

Get out of the habit of grazing in front of the TV, eating on the run, or nibbling at your desk. Sit at the table to eat your meal, turn off the TV or laptop, and savour your food. You'll enjoy your meal more, your digestion will be better, and you'll probably eat less overall.

 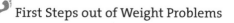

7. Eat first what you should, then what you would

Fill up on healthy foods that will nourish your body. After that, you can have a treat if you feel like it. But reach for the sugary indulgences first and you won't have any appetite for the nutritious foods your body needs.

What people say...

When I weighed 15st 5lb (98kg), I lived my life around food and was always looking forward to my next meal or snack. If I was feeling down, I'd cheer myself up with a bag of crisps or a slice of cake. Now, I eat to live rather than live to eat. Life is about planning what I can do with my day, not what I'm going to eat. I still go to the gym regularly and have loads of energy. I love dressing up in pretty outfits and bright colours. I'm bubbly and happy and my husband loves the new me – I'm never going back to the old version!

Janine, 29, now 10st 8lb (67kg) and size UK12

Over to you!

Congratulations! You've reached your target and are now in a healthy weight range for your height. And by continuing to live a healthy, active life, you'll be able to keep the weight off for good. Be ready with a strategy if the pounds start to creep on again, but don't let your weight become an obsession – it's held you back from making the most of your life for long enough. Now you can look and feel your best, enjoy being fit and active, and know that you've given your body its best chance of staying healthy. It's time to enjoy being you!

For the family

Losing weight is a big challenge for anyone. It requires a major change in terms of cooking and eating, which can also affect other members of the household. It means finding time to incorporate more activity into daily life. Your family member has decided the time has come to tackle their weight problem, and this is bound to have a knock-on effect on the rest of the family.

You're probably very familiar with the negative effects of being overweight, which may have affected your loved one for years or even decades. Their health may be suffering. They may struggle with daily activities such as walking reasonable distances or running around after the children. They may feel self-conscious or distressed about their appearance and have low self-esteem. If they're your partner, this may well affect your relationship. So no doubt you're keen to encourage your loved one to become healthier and enjoy a better quality of life by losing the excess weight – and you'll reap the rewards, too.

On the other hand, you may have watched your family member try to shape up in the past. You may be cynical and wonder if this latest attempt will be any more successful than previous efforts. And, yes, the likelihood is they will sometimes struggle to stay on track. But if you want them to succeed this time, there are ways you can help them.

Be willing to adapt your eating habits

If you eat together as a couple or family, being prepared to adjust your eating habits a little will make a huge difference to your loved one being able to stick to a healthy diet. It doesn't mean you have to live on lettuce leaves or give up all your favourite foods. But if they want to experiment with creating low-fat versions of your usual meals, or try out new, healthier recipes, it will help them tremendously if other family members are open to something different. Having to cook and eat something different from the rest of the household makes it much tougher. If you're the main cook in the house, making an effort to try new, healthier recipes is a wonderful way to show your family member you love them and are supporting their efforts. You might even lose a few pounds yourself.

If the cupboards are normally full of crisps, biscuits, and chocolate, it will be more difficult for your loved one to avoid temptation. If you can see your way to having fewer of these foods around the house, or keeping them in a less accessible place and not indulging too much in front of your family member, it will be easier for them to stick to their plan.

Be prepared to join in activities

As well as an exercise plan, your loved one may be hoping to include more activity in their daily life. This may

For the family 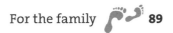 **89**

include going walking or cycling instead of sitting in front of the TV, starting a new hobby such as tennis, or taking the children swimming at the weekends. Being willing to adapt your own leisure time to become more active – or perhaps looking after the children to allow your family member to get out and about – will help them boost their fitness levels. Being more active will also benefit your own health and well-being, so everyone wins.

Give them extra time

It's difficult to concentrate on your own needs if you're always busy and stressed out. It will help your family member if they have a few less worries and a bit more time to themselves. Can you take on any extra responsibilities in the home to give them a chance to relax and take care of themselves? Could you look after the children a couple of evenings a week so your loved one can go to the gym or for a run? Are you willing to adapt your routine so they can get an early night a couple of times a week? Anything that lowers their stress levels and gives them some "me time" will make them more likely to achieve their weight-loss goal.

Keep encouraging them

As time goes on, your family member may lose motivation to persevere with their diet and exercise regime, especially if the weight is coming off slowly. Your support and encouragement will make all the difference. If their enthusiasm for eating healthily is waning, prompt them with reminders of why they want to get into shape. If they're not in the mood to go to an exercise class, remind them how good they'll feel afterwards. Encourage them to stay on track by pointing out how far they've come already. Boost their self-esteem by complimenting them on their improving shape – perhaps even offer to buy them a new outfit to show off their figure. And if they fall off the wagon, persuade them not to give up altogether and to get back on track straight away. They're much more likely to succeed with you as their cheerleader.

 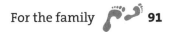

Useful resources

Recommended reading

- *The Calorie, Carb and Fat Bible 2011* by Juliette Kellow, Lyndel Costain and Laurence Beeken (Weight Loss Resources, 2011)

- *Collins Gem Calorie Counter* (Collins, 2010)

- *Restaurant Calorie Counter for Dummies* by Rosanne Rust and Meri Raffetto (John Wiley & Sons, 2011)

- *Easy GI Diet* by Helen Foster (Hamlyn, 2008)

- *Fitness for Life Manual* by Matt Roberts (Dorling Kindersley, 2011)

- *The Portion Teller* by Lisa R. Young (Broadway Books, 2005)

Online resources

For an online BMI calculator and other helpful resources, visit: www.bmi-calculator.net

For an online calorie counter, recipes, and online food and exercise diaries, visit www.weightlossresources.co.uk

For the Diet Plate range of products, visit www.thedietplate.com

For the latest research and advice from experts in your country, visit the following websites:

UK: www.nhs.uk/change4life and www.nationalobesityforum.org.uk

USA: www.nutrition.gov

Canada: www.hc-sc.gc.ca

Australia: www.nutritionaustralia.org

New Zealand: www.nutritionfoundation.org.nz

Slimming clubs

Slimming World: www.slimmingworld.com (international)

Weight Watchers: www.weightwatchers.com (international)

Rosemary Conley Diet and Fitness Clubs: www.rosemaryconley.com (UK)

Eating disorders

For help with eating disorders, and contact information for support organizations around the world, read *First Steps out of Eating Disorders* by Dr Kate Middleton and Dr Jane Smith (Lion Hudson, 2010)

Diet diary chart

	Breakfast	Lunch	Dinner	Snacks	Cals/Fat	Exercise
Monday						
Tuesday						
Wednesday						
Thursday						
Friday						
Saturday						
Sunday						

First Steps out of Weight Problems

Progress chart

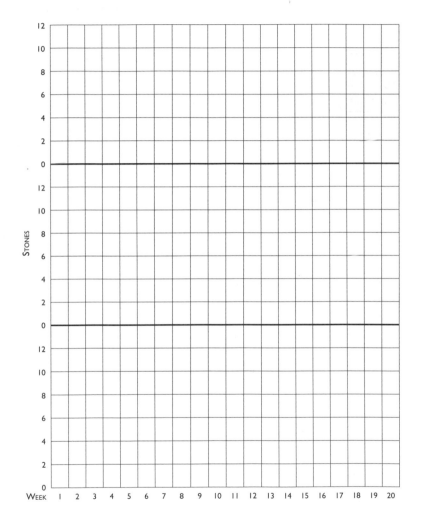

STONES

12																				
10																				
8																				
6																				
4																				
2																				
0																				

WEEK 1 2 3 4 5 6 7 8 9 10 11 12 13 14 15 16 17 18 19 20

 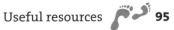

International dress sizes
UK clothing sizes are used throughout the book.
Equivalent clothing sizes for the USA, Canada, Australia
and New Zealand are as follows:

UK	USA/Canada	Australia/ New Zealand
8	6	10
10	8	12
12	10	14
14	12	16
16	14	18
18	16	20
20	18	22
22	20	24
24	22	26
26	24	28
28	26	30

Stones/pounds conversion
Weights are given in stones/pounds and kilograms. For
those more familiar with measuring weight in pounds
only, here is a quick guide:

Stones	Pounds
1	14
8	112
9	126
10	140
11	154
12	168
13	182
14	196
15	210
16	224
17	238
18	252
19	266
20	280
21	294